FROM BLACK CABBING
TO BLACKOUTS

Ian Starkey

Published by New Generation Publishing in 2016

ISBN 978-1-78507-820-0

www.newgeneration-publishing.com

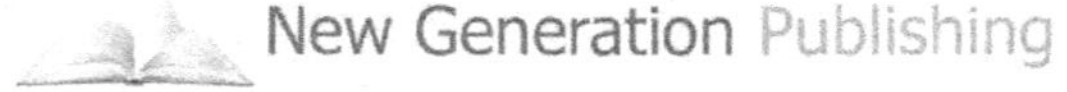

DEDICATIONS

*Written with a huge thanks to Mum and Dad
for never giving up on me.*

In memory of

*John Andrews
Tracey Andrews
Kevin Shipsey
Rob Prior
Mark Thompson (ginger)
Vic Richardson*

All taken far too early and will never be forgotten.

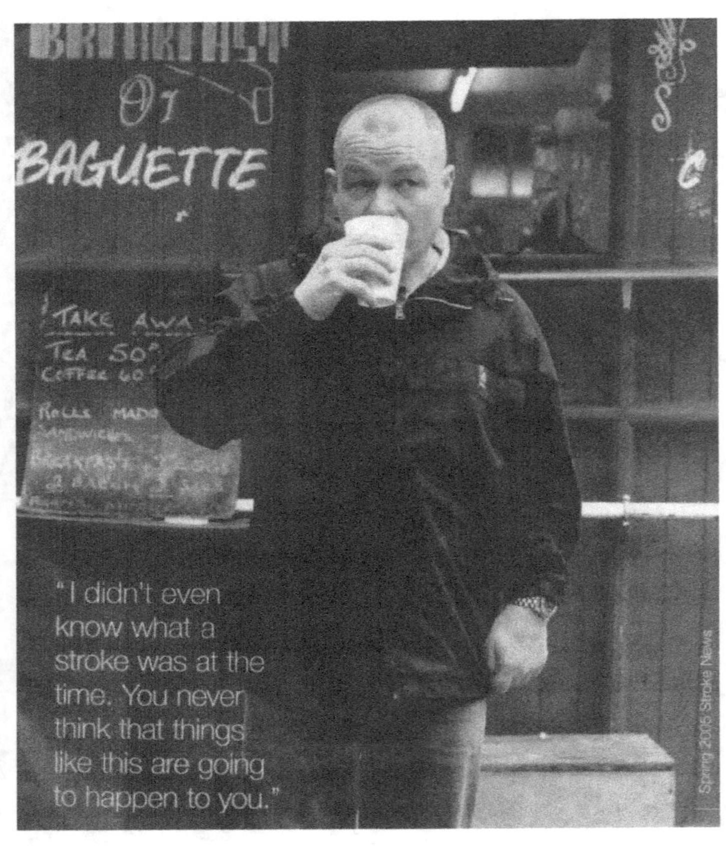

**"WHEN A MAN IS TIRED OF LONDON,
HE IS TIRED OF LIFE."**

INTRODUCTION

Come and join me on a forty-year journey where I will try to look at the lighter side of driving a black taxi around London for fifteen years, with a selection of some of the interesting characters I had the pleasure of bumping into and situations I found myself in.

Supporting Chelsea Football club through thick and thin home and abroad from being nearly bankrupt to the financial heavyweights they are today, whilst also travelling overseas to watch the England football team by motorcycle, all financed by earning a living driving a black cab, throw in an array of other typical lads adventures home and abroad.

Much of it regrettably forgotten due to drink and late nights all leading up to a life changing situation, for which at no time will I look for any praise or sympathy.

AUTHOR BIOGRAPHY

Ian Starkey was born into a stable family in the early sixties. He attended the local junior and comprehensive schools, where he found that he preferred football to academia. His father provided well for the family by running a small, fairly successful, building firm. Starkey's father discouraged his sons from following in his footsteps.

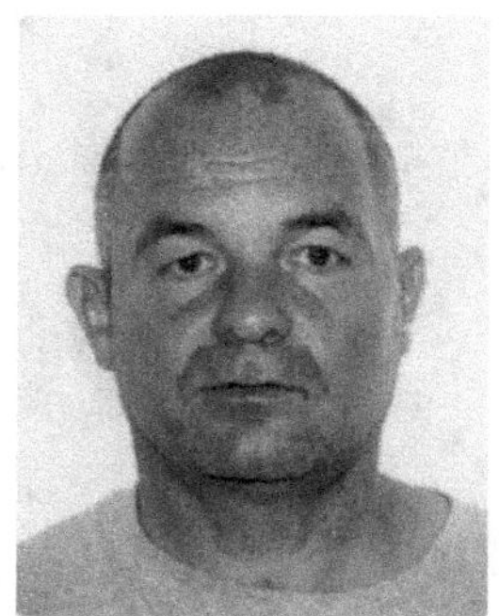

Upon leaving school, following a series of unfulfilling and limiting jobs, Starkey trained to become a London taxi driver. He found himself enjoying his work immensely, travelling around the world, and indulging in an extravagant lifestyle. He immersed himself in the music, culture and fashion of the late seventies and early eighties. During this time, he had a keen interest in football, supporting Chelsea F.C. and England, often travelling to away matches on his motorcycle.

After driving for 15 years Starkey's life changed drastically when he suffered a severe stroke. The next three years tested Starkey to his limits with further issues, resulting in blackouts. Struggling to keep his license he was unable to live the life he loved so much.

Starkey's positive attitude still shines through despite everything. Seeing himself as a stroke survivor, rather than a victim, convinced him to change his lifestyle and document his experience. He can still be seen wandering around the capital, although now with a slight limp, with the same positive attitude.

CONTENTS

Sometime this century, whilst on a solo drink in Camden, came an uninvited quote from a fellow lost solo female barfly:

"The eyes are the key to the soul, young man, and yours tell the tale of a life that has played many parts and perhaps you need to carefully select in which direction to head now."

Part 1

Early Days and Football

It all started with a completely normal north-east London home life, happily married parents, older brother, food on the table every, night relatives and neighbours all normal – no crazy alcoholics or middle-aged hippies to influence me.

Attended local junior school and then on to senior comprehensive; have kept in touch with a few people but only those that I wanted to (Friends Reunited and Facebook (my personal opinion of these websites is if we haven't spoken for thirty-five years would we have anything to say now?).

Education came to an end in May 1979 no more classrooms for me (as I always knew best); apprenticeships – no way, just a couple of dead-end office jobs and waste of time glorified bits of labouring work whatever offered the most pay, schools career advice had obviously not sunk in.

Final School Report:

'Should and could have done better.'

FOOTBALL

Football has always been one of the great passions of my life, playing when younger whilst always a regular spectator – won't start off by saying where we lived there was no grass or I had no football boots or that by the time I hit my teens a few professional clubs were interested but due to me being a bit of a maverick and too heavy on the drink they lost interest (anyone who knows me would know this to be complete fantasy).

However watching football home and abroad following Chelsea and England I have had some of the best times of my life, completely misinterpreted by some tabloids.

The camaraderie between the lads is hard to explain unless you were there.

It may seem strange to some that I come from north-east London and follow Chelsea.

HOW IT STARTED

Watching the 1970 F.A. cup final on TV, being a black and white set, Chelsea in dark kits and Leeds in white kits seeing my intense interest it was quickly explained to me that the team in dark kits came from London and therefore one day I may be able to go and watch them live.

FROM MILLMOOR TO MOSCOW

Baptism day arrived when in the fifth round of the F.A. cup in 1972, second division Leyton Orient drew the mighty Chelsea at Orient's Brisbane Road ground in Leyton.

Dad took me along and of course things went to plan as Chelsea stormed into a two-goal lead; however on a mudbath of a pitch Orient struck back with three to knock Chelsea out of the competition.

Let's just call it a bad day at the office, oh boy was I to experience a few more of those over the next thirty years!

This was the beginning of my journey, throughout the late seventies. I was of course still at school whilst still playing but did manage to jump on the train across town to Stamford Bridge and attend some away games when possible.

By the time the early eighties arrived the club had really fallen from grace and now in the old second division with serious financial difficulties facing the club for the second time, green bins were positioned around the forecourt of the ground in order to collect spare change for the 'save the bridge' fund.

At this point I had started to travel away on a regular basis with my three local friends (Darrell, usually much appreciated driver; Harry and Jason). I was also getting to get to know a few of the other regular away-day lads.

Terrace fashion had changed – the old seventies skinhead-look had virtually disappeared to be replaced by designer casual outfits, personally I always tried to dress smart but not go over the top still wearing similar button-down collar shirts to this day.

One of my most memorable trips ever came in October 1981 when I embarked on a solo Ian day out to Rotherham.

Millmoor was the name of Rotherham's ground where Chelsea had a nightmare, getting thrashed six nil.

Nowadays rival fans accuse us of being glory hunters who have jumped on the successes bandwagon.

There is always a dispute at football about who are proper fans – as far as I'm concerned, the fans who were on that terrace with me on that dismal day in Yorkshire you are proper Chelsea and I salute every one of you.

From here onwards my personal journey took me the width of Britain from the south coast to the north-east via the Midlands, north west and Wales.

In 1995 our trips further afield started when Chelsea qualified for Europe taking us to a whole new dimension leading up to an unforgettable trip I was in attendance for when we lost the 2008 champions league final in Moscow.

My loyalty and commitment can never be questioned and if in those dark days in the early eighties we had gone bankrupt, ending up in the blue square/conference league, I'm sure I would still be a season-ticket holder as I am at present attending all home games and as many away domestic and European as possible.

This superb adventure continues, still enjoying every minute of the ride (whilst fully realising the bubble could burst at any time).

Personally I don't think we can thank Roman Abramavich (club owner) enough for providing the finances to take us to this level – umpteen domestic cups, three league titles with one double thrown in and to be mentioned later in book perhaps the best trip of my life a champions league title win.

Back to that completely different era of the eighties –, some of the players who wore the blue shirt in those days ended up studying for the 'knowledge' (learning the streets of London to become black taxi drivers when their career was over) not something you can imagine happening to any of the current squad but a path my own life was to follow.

With no particular career path mapped out in the early eighties, the legendary cheap jaunts abroad started – Majorca, Ibiza, Corfu and various other Med destinations. Tried my hand with a few of the other lads, handing out promotional tickets for nightclubs whilst on the beach during the day, but let's face it the c.v. for the job is far more suited to girls who perhaps could have found alternative employment in a lap-dancing club rather than lads who look straight off the football terraces.

January 1983 I headed off to Israel to work on a kibbutz (farm), but instead of picking apples in the sun found myself positioned in a hot factory injecting chickens against cholera who took great delight in crapping all over me.

Returning home earlier than planned was probably the wrong decision (isn't hindsight a fine thing). But this turned out to be a turning point in my life as I was now in my early twenties and really needed to sort myself out, therefore deciding to sign on for the knowledge train to become a London black taxi driver.

This entailed learning every street in London by riding around on a small motorbike with a map board attached between the handlebars remembering all important buildings and how to get from one to another by the quickest route, whilst enrolling in a school to revise and repeat these routes parrot-fashion in the afternoons with other knowledge boys and girls.

Overall after a bit of messing about here and there I passed out (receiving my much coveted green badge in January 1987).

Luckily for me throughout the knowledge I lived with my parents, subsidising myself with a bit of courier work as I had got to adore my little Honda c 90 whilst most of the other pupils hated theirs. ('Won't say I never came off, was even knocked off'), with the culprit disappearing up the Harrow Road without a glance in his mirror although fully aware of his misdemeanour.

Getting soaked to the skin became second nature, which was nothing new as I did have a bit of history with motorcycling having owned a 50 cc M Z moped enabling me to travel the last five months to senior school and back instead of using the bus; luckily for me only about three miles but too far to walk at sixteen. You were legally allowed to do this even though I had no idea of road etiquette or proper understanding of the Highway Code, as at the time no training was required.

Filter lights – ignore them and just go, and I certainly wasn't the only one must have been like the children's seventies cartoon THE WACCY RACES!

Whilst on the knowledge, another major pastime cropped up – I had been bitten by the motorcycle bug, enjoying the freedom so much on my little c90 even taking my test enabling me to upgrade to any size of bike I desired but opted for a Honda 650 Silverwing, a touring bike with full luggage space.

This gave me a whole new way of following Chelsea and even took it to Germany to follow the England football team in the 1988 European championships. Another classic motorcycle adventure embarked upon was in 1997 – a solo trip up the east coast of Australia.

I TRAVELLED LIGHT AND I TRAVELLED ALONE.

Part 2

Wearing The Green Badge

As a newly qualified cabbie, in January 1987 I took to my new life like a duck to water.

There have been other books written about the cab trade, covering all the usual aspects from the strict laws of the Public Carriage Office, who run the trade and test the knowledge boys to how drivers are allowed to urinate over the back wheel if they are concealed by a cloak and carrying a barrel of hay, the journey of evolution from horse-drawn carriages to the smart Mercedes Vito cabs available today.

This is a short story of my time in the cab trade, throwing in a few of my favourite tales and how it affected and changed my life.

As a London taxi driver you do find yourself stereotyped but I was determined to buck this trend by only speaking when spoken to (not being the particular chatty-type anyway) found this easy.

If I meet any trainee cabbies (knowledge pupils) nowadays the only advice I can offer is to avoid discussions on politics, religion, or football and try to make them realise they will be called upon to play many parts such as restaurant critic, shares expert whilst offering marital advice and other health issues whilst being fully bilingual.

There are four questions I was most commonly asked by passengers and friends who are not in the trade:

Number 1 (and most common)

How much do you cab drivers earn?

Answer, easy one that – NONE OF YOUR BUSINESS!

Number 2

Did you ever sleep with or get any offers from any of the girls you picked up?

Answer, no.

Number 3

Did you ever have a couple having sex in the back?

Answer, no.

Number 4

Who was your most famous passenger?

Many an actor/actress, MPs and a lot of public figures use cabs – a common occurrence when plying for hire (looking for a passenger) on the capital's busy streets.

I have never really understood autograph books and consider it rude to invade other people's privacy (treat others as you would like to be treated yourself) and never wanted to admit recognizing anyone, won't say the temptation wasn't there to ask Joan Collins or Dame Judi Dench if I had seen them somewhere before.

By 1988 I had come to realise it was more profitable to join a radio circuit, giving me two options of picking up fares – pre-booked radio jobs and street hails as well.

One Saturday night heading down the West Cromwell Road a job was offered on the radio in SW5 Earls Court area; being the nearest available cab I was allocated the job. When the details appeared on my work screen I noticed the passenger-to-be Mr Freddy Freestone; at the time Chelsea had a reserve goalkeeper named Roger Freestone whom the fans nicknamed Freddy (not a household name by any means in footballing terms.

Having accepted the job on arrival at the address behind a large, white, brick wall although near to the ground, I thought this to be an extremely plush residence for a reserve goalkeeper and also a bit strange to use a terrace nickname for booking cabs, remembering this was the late eighties and football was different then. I was a bit shocked when our second-choice goalkeeper came out with two large mates and sat in the middle of them, whilst not appearing particularly tall for a goalkeeper.

Once p.o.b. (Passenger On Board), the lads requested Queensway, just the other side of Hyde Park. One of them made a bit of small talk with me whilst I did converse briefly with Roger who seemed really quiet – when he spoke the others listened as he had a certain aura about him.

It would have been rude to turn round and stare but whilst glancing in the mirror the penny had started to drop, I may have seen Roger Freestone play at Stamford Bridge and not properly recognized him, but I had been fortunate enough to see my current passenger take Wembley Stadium by storm at Live Aid – it was unbelievably the legendary FREDDIE MERCURY.

AND IT DOESN'T GET MUCH MORE FAMOUS THAN THAT!

The morning after Freddie died I had to retrace the steps of my most famous journey and tried to drive as near as possible to LOGAN MEWS which was packed solid with people paying tribute and which I now believe to be a Freddie museum.

LONDON'S INTRESTING MIX OF CHRACTERS.

Every year I carried hundreds of passengers, ranging from top city businessman to cleaners, professional sportsmen, actors, and an assortment of media types, whilst some of the most memorable were streetwise types who only seemed to appear when darkness fell, amongst them chancers spivs and girls who worked in the oldest profession in the world. Certain areas of the capital at night seemed to attract characters who you just could not invent but it had a certain vibe which makes London special and I really enjoyed being part of it (well as much as you could whilst working).

Once my cab was on the road I never knew what to expect – some of the tourists' requests (a book in itself) ranged from an American couple asking if I could arrange an introduction to Eric Clapton, to an Australian girl enquiring why the strange looking old brick building located on the river by Tower Hill had men in dresses (Beefeaters) positioned outside. Throw in remarkable destinations asked for in all seriousness, such as "can you take us to Den and Angie's pub in Albert Square please?"

Over the next few pages let me introduce you to some of my favourite/most memorable situations that stand in the memory and are as much a part of London as the red buses and phone boxes – no offence intended if any of you are still out there, which I very much doubt as some of these events occurred as long as Twenty Five years ago or more. And I certainly wouldn't recognise you again.

ALERT SAVILE ROW POLICE STATION!

One midsummer afternoon I received a job to pick up from one of London's most plush jewellery shops in Old Bond Street – for once being lucky enough to find a parking meter located directly outside the entrance to wait for my passenger who was not yet anywhere to be seen, therefore enabling me to leave the cab for a brief glimpse in the window/covered lobby at the glistening goodies on show. Also looking was a slightly younger guy sporting a tracksuit, probably early twenties; we exchanged pleasantries like a pair of school kids as we were both admirers of the superb range of watches on show – Rolex, Brietling, Tag and various others I had never heard of.

On returning to the cab, after another short wait about fifteen minutes overall, my passenger boarded – a smartly dressed middle-aged woman and we set off to our destination.

"Sorry for keeping you waiting, driver, but we had a bit of a security scare and were about to phone Savile Row police station to make them aware of the situation." Can't say I personally noticed any ram-raiding trucks cruising down Bond Street.

Then she continued, "had a couple of suspicious characters on the premises – youngish guy and older shaven-headed shifty-looking guy, probably a proper Fagin never done an honest day's work between them, you know the types."

As we got caught in some heavy traffic she started fidgeting nervously in her handbag pulling out her small vanity mirror to pretend she was adjusting her perfectly applied make-up to avoid any eye contact with me in order to cover up her blatant identity mistake.

LESSONS IN LIFE FROM MY TEENAGE DREAM GIRL

When picking up passengers I used to play a silly game of giving them lookalike names in my head – Ronald Reagan, Marilyn Monroe, Rupert Bear and Doctor Who all travelled in my taxi.

She strode with a real purpose out of a store in Oxford Street, the years had been good to her, hailing me down confidently sporting trademark denim jacket and tight leather jeans – it had to be Suzi Quatro.

In my teens I remember having a real crush on the raunchy rock chic. Suzi lookalike requested Camden, whilst heading through the heavy traffic in Tottenham Court Road I was quietly humming I hope "can the can and devilgate drive" (famous Suzi Quatro 1970's hits) if my passenger could hear me she must have thought this driver is deluded as she did bear a splitting double for the classic 70's rocker.

On reaching our destination in Camden, having come to a halt, the meter clicked up another twenty pence (for those of you who don't know taxi meters run on a time and motion this was not some scam I was operating).

Suzi lookalike had stepped out and was preparing to pay me through the passenger window, when I requested the original fare not including the last twenty pence.

Suzi slapped her leather-clad thigh and placed the correct fare in my hand leaving me with this last remark "take this as a lesson and don't you ever do that again as NICE GUYS COME LAST."

Never a truer word spoken

A lesson I have since taken on board.

LOOK INTO MY EYES

Lunchtime is usually a major part of the cabbie's day. Located around London there are a number of green huts similar to old Victorian-style police booths; these huts are where many drivers meet for lunch (at least one of them I believe to be a listed building).

This was not for me although I did pop in occasionally (full of characters, and taxi folklore legend has it that Frank Sinatra once enjoyed a fry-up in one of these establishments).

Many of my favourite lunchtimes were spent parked up on the end of a taxi rank, sitting in the back of my cab especially on a nice summer day with the back door open.

One particularly hot day I had grabbed myself a sandwich and coffee, got myself well settled in, normal position sitting on the backseat feet up on pull-down spring seat.

When all of a sudden to my horror a woman had collapsed directly beside my cab and was finding difficulty in getting back on her feet. Of course I assisted, jumping out and helping her on her way.

On returning to my cab, having finished my lunch about ten minutes later, I decided to return to work gathered up my empty sandwich packet and coffee cup to discard in the bin.

But alas no moneybag (the most important part of the cabbie's kit contains everything) jumped out of the cab looked underneath and on the roof in case I had put it there by mistake, did a quick Basil Fawlty (jumped up and down on the pavement) by now coming to accept what had happened.

Luckily the keys were not in my bag; locked the cab up and walked to the nearest phone box in the naive hope that some good Samaritan had handed my bag in.

As I had no change, dialled a free 'lost property' number where the person on the other end asked all the correct questions – "contents of bag" to which I answered "bankcard, full cash float around fifty pounds, A.A. and library cards, Chelsea season ticket" – could have done without the next sarcastic comment "the way they are playing, probably done you a favour."

When I related my tale to one of my pals who drives a train, he told me of a similar tale he had heard doing the rounds on the underground of a woman hypnotising people and stealing from them.

Looking back on my damsel in distress I have to say when she was on the pavement her eyes did seem transfixed into mine whilst her heavy mascara and over-the-top bright silver necklaces were a superb distraction, a back-handed compliment really as you were good at what you did, although I do not think you were the alleged underground trickster and had me under your hypnotic spell.

Getting everything reinstated from my money bag proved a real hassle – one of the strangest things, a mobile phone line opened in my name with a bill arriving for worldwide calls but luckily I never had to settle up.

TALES OF A SOHO PHONE BOX

By the mid-nineties mobiles were the 'must have' thing and regularly being left in the back of my cab. Suddenly I would hear a strange ringtone of which if I could find had no idea how to answer; this would quickly be followed by an urgent request broadcast on my work radio to immediately return the handset to an important client from one of our accounts who thought they may have left their phone in the cab.

Personally I did not possess one of these nuisance things until this century; when admitting this I was virtually accused of being a leper or creature from outer space "why don't you want to give me your number?"

Twenty-five years ago if you arranged to meet someone you turned up on time but it is now seems to be acceptable to notify someone you will be late by text and leave them waiting around.

Mobiles were also responsible for another social role reversal – if you wanted to spark up a conversation with a girl you used to offer to buy her a drink, come the mobile revolution girls would approach you with the enquiry "got any credit on your phone, mate?"

Not being an owner of a handset, one night in the early nineties around Soho I desperately needed to make a call whilst working, having tried the first couple of old red traditional phone boxes which tourists adore – they were either out of order, or reeking of urine (very quaint British custom).

Finally I found one of those grey metal things with no front door offering no privacy whatsoever; plastered all over the ceiling and back walls were prostitutes' business cards. Having sorted my friend's number out I searched my pockets for twenty and fifty pence pieces – perhaps this was a different kind of sterling or mine were the wrong shape? I stood there leaning against the phone balancing the wire between the handset and my ear probably hoping the coin slot may repair itself. All of a sudden a guy approached, rather too close for comfort, leant over my crouched shoulder and stuck a business card just above me (Scandinavian babe, local, all services). In no uncertain terms I pointed out that I was using this piece of telecom's finest, and with that he disappeared off into this vibrant part of town.

Welcome to the festive season.

When you cannot switch radio stations or browse around a shop without hearing Slade Wizard and Greg Lake (those classic Christmas hits) every cabbie has a tale to tell.

The last Thursday before Christmas, slowly driving past one of London's famous city livery halls where a couple hailed me down who were suitably attired for a part in Downtown Abbey.

Acting in a most gentlemanly manner, the chap opens the rear door whilst his date steps in alone. As she gets settled in he requests the destination and pays the fare in advance with this remark, "take care, especially over the speed bumps as my little hunny is a bit delicate having injured her back at a pilates session."

We set off on our journey getting caught in a bit of traffic as the girl enquires, "Driver, how do these back windows come down?" my only suggestion being try the switch that states "these windows are electronically operated" by now beginning to think that my passenger is trying to practise her pilates breathing technique out loud. We do make it to her house where, as we are approaching she casually states, "why is it at these corporate functions you are not warned that sushi and red wine do not mix?"

Enough said!

Of course that night's 'work shift' was brought to an early end as the aroma of washed-out sick would not have been a great encouragement for further passengers.

But credit where credit's due, she did send me a cheque in the new year towards my taxi cleaning expenses.

Part 3

Twenty-Five Years Living Life to the Full and a Couple of Unforgettable Trips.

ENLISTMENT FOR THE BOOZE BATTLEFIELD

From 1979 to 2003 I served in the weekend booze regiment visiting watering holes throughout London and Britain whilst sometimes being called on duty further afield. Many members of this force excelled in the language of lager and talking complete and utter shit – you never knew where you might end up and whenever I see down-and-outs on a park bench I think "there for the grace of God goes I."

Slightly older people often use the phrase "if you can remember the sixties you weren't really there" – don't tell me this won't be said about the seventies, eighties and this century as well.

In the mid-to-late seventies, disco music was at its height but never really did it for me preferring The Jam, Rolling Stones, Ian Dury and The Blockheads and Squeeze, all of which apart from The Jam I have been lucky enough to see live.

Whilst being in attendance for most of these events plus other memorable occasions such as Scotland 0 England 2 at Hampden Park; Germany 1 England 5 in Munich; many big Chelsea games; the original Live Aid along with many other outdoor festivals I have to admit being under the booze influence and ask myself did I really enjoy them?

But I wouldn't change a thing!

Once Pandora's box was open there was no telling where the journey would take you.

My lifestyle was never directly diagnosed for future health problems (to be explained two chapters on probably more natural issues).

THE DUCK POND MAN

My new occupation as a taxi driver financed some superb trips all around the Med, Cuba and Thailand whilst two of the most memorable already briefly mentioned were on two wheels (by motorcycle) – in 1997 a trip up the east coast of Australia from Sydney to Byron Bay.

Whilst my favourite and most memorable was when two of my favourite pastimes came together in June 1988 when the England football team competed in the European championships in Germany.

Firstly I was successful in my application for tickets and had my trusty steed Honda 650 Silverwing to get me there.

Next came accommodation – bought myself a tent of which having had a dummy run to assemble in my mum's garden didn't seem able to master even though I was twenty-five at the time. My mum had to remark "remember when you wouldn't join the scouts, if you had that would be a piece of cake."

When I did set off on a glorious day in late May I already knew this was going to be something special. Pulling onto the A12 bound for Harwich, my heavy-laden two-wheeled companion all set for adventure, I was singing my head off "king of the road" (can't beat a bit of Sinatra/Dean Martin). Motorcycle travel is special, just you and the elements right on the edge, other bikers and complete strangers give you a friendly wave.

Approaching Harwich the salty sea air fills your nostrils, filing onto the ferry bound for the Hook of Holland myself and the deckhand make small talk as he secures my bike with a sturdy rope, "why don't you fly or catch a train?"

"If I tried to explain you wouldn't understand."

If I remember correctly the night crossing took about eight hours; disembarking on Dutch soil the next morning it seemed strange following road signs in a different language.

On arrival in Amsterdam my first night was to be spent in a low budget hotel which I had stayed in once before. On check-in the manager gave me strict orders to lock my bike in an underground car park.

Amsterdam at night at that time was a strange place, prostitutes sitting in windows offering their services and all sorts of strange characters wandering the streets, however this shouldn't be misinterpreted as there was also a great aroma of coffee in the air from the many small legendary coffee shops.

Leaving Amsterdam the next morning needing to head north for Germany, following my tank map, I was pulling up in the street and asking people the way to Dusseldorf (no satellite navigation in those days) heading out of Holland I saw my first windmill. Crossing the border early evening into Germany, a strange feeling as on the autobahns there are no speed limits and people seem to drive like maniacs although they do show utmost respect to motorcycles especially those with foreign number plates.

Darkness was slightly falling as I pulled onto the designated football campsite, when all of a sudden that feeling that every biker knows hit me, my back wheel was sliding but to top it there was water creeping up my boots.

OH NO! I have slid into the edge of a pond and my trusty steed is over, whilst petrified ducks are squawking in fear. That pond should have been roped off – so much for German efficiency.

Other campers rushed to assist yes I've arrived, with help bike out, totally wet tent laid out to dry.

This again was a solo Ian trip that night I walked down to the string of bars in town which were packed with fans from the campsite English and Dutch where I was greeted with the same words from the few campers who had witnessed my tumble "there's the guy who fell in the duck pond, come and join us".

Over the next few weeks I enjoyed a fantastic time even though England got knocked out earlier than we all hoped.

Throughout the years I have always kept my interest in two wheels, hiring a similar Honda to follow England at Euro 2000 in Belgium, whilst nowadays switching to scooters even attending the isle of Wight scooter rally a couple of times where every August bank holiday thousands of scooters descend on the island for a party even though I arrive by train I am not as sad that I walk around with a crash helmet under my arm.

APRÈS SKI TO A&E

Getting away from football trips I did have other interests, ever since the last couple of years at senior school having always been a keen skier trying to attend as often as possible financed by my new taxi-driving lifestyle.

In March 2003, myself and three good friends enjoyed a mad week on the slopes of France, late nights, not producing the most stylish performances the following mornings. During the final run down the piste Saturday afternoon I took a bit of a tumble on the junior (learner slopes) banging my head in the process in the soft powdery snow – nothing I hadn't encountered before but a bit strange for someone who had probably been skiing on and off for fifteen years, but the mountain can often spring an unexpected surprise – getting up and dusting myself off at the time thinking no more of it.

Sunday afternoon we flew into Stanstead airport where my cab was parked and I drove myself and three weary passengers home about twenty miles away, a good time had been had by all.

Monday 24th March, back to work as normal, completed the daytime shift in the cab, parking up early evening near my central London gym where I usually took part in an organised circuit class three times per week.

During the class I tripped on a crash mat and vaguely remember the instructor insisting on phoning for an ambulance as he seemed to think that I had blacked out on my feet.

When I regained consciousness, apparently the next morning surrounded by medical staff, I was informed that I was in the University College Hospital in central London having never been in hospital before, the nearest to this particular one to drop passengers off.

By now I was thinking, you have really done it this time my old son, realising that I seemed to have some kind of paralysis down my left side and was slurring when attempting to speak.

Then came the bombshell as the chief consultant approached my bed to inform me that I had suffered a stroke. Having no idea what that was he explained to me an interruption of the blood flow to the brain depriving it of oxygen and in my case injuring the part which controls the left-hand side of the body, not to be confused with a heart attack – a misconception I have regularly came across since.

For the next week I was wheelchair-bound, being unable to put any weight on my left leg or use my left arm.

As soon as possible I was transferred from an acute brain injury ward to a rehabilitation ward at the National

Hospital in Queen Square in London where I stayed for two months.

I can never praise the staff enough at these hospitals for their dedication, professional treatment, and understanding in what were strange out-of-the blue circumstances. Some of my fellow patients were suffering from guillain barre syndrome, a neurological disorder in which the body's own immune system attacks their own nervous system, also Parkinson's and different stages of multiple sclerosis.

For all of us being assisted to the toilet and having your food cut up was an embarrassing life-changing situation.

My discharge came after two months and I still have physio right up to today; however it is all a bit of a blur as it was thirteen years ago.

The cause of my stroke was never really discovered, maybe a concoction of both high cholesterol and high blood pressure neither of which I was aware.

I also doubt if the excessive banana shots après ski or occasional weekend boozing previous helped.

At this point I was duty bound to tell the authorities who run the London taxi trade (the Public Carriage Office) and the D.V.L.A. of my situation which meant handing my London green taxi badge back.

Of course this was one of the hardest things I ever had to do as I had tried so hard all those years ago to pass the knowledge and get one.

QUEEN ELIZABETH FOUNDATION

Whilst an inpatient at Queen Square Hospital my occupational therapist (Zoe Martin) informed me about the Queen Elizabeth Foundation Mobility Centre which provides an extensive training programme for people with disabilities who wish to learn or relearn to drive and gives advice about car adaptions to suit particular needs.

Having managed to gain a sponsor through the hospital (big thanks to Zoe and sponsor the lady Samaritans) I was accepted.

In November 2003 an appointment was made. When entering the waiting area of the centre at Carshalton Beeches in Surrey, I was amazed at the impressive photos on the walls of former pupils who had overcome their disabilities to regain independence.

On view out of the window the staff could be seen patiently taking trainees through their paces.

Then to my delight I was summoned; having already checked my lifestyle and medical history thoroughly my personal assessment began, first orthotic to check that my eyesight was still up to driving, next orientation and perceptual tests followed by a static rig which really examined my reactions.

Following all this for the first time in seven months I climbed behind the wheel of a Nissan Micra and set off around the mobility centre's private track which offers bends, hills, and junctions on an old hospital road network.

The Nissan Micra was fitted with infra-red controls which control anything you normally activate with your left hand and allowed one-hand steering.

It was strange to get used to at first as I found myself veering to the left-hand side of the road, but in the afternoon my instructor considered me safe enough to take out on the road, of course accompanied by him.

The conclusion of my first day at the Q.E.F. was to return in January for a further lesson, which of course I did and proved a major step, resulting in the mobility centre giving me the all clear to drive an adapted vehicle.

Following this I had to apply to the D.V.L.A. for a licence with adapted steering wheel controls when the anniversary of my stroke arose – which they agreed to.

But the next stage was always going to be a huge hurdle – proving to Public Carriage Office that I was fit to taxi passengers around.

Following a doctor's report, hospital and mobility centre report, seventeen months after suffering a stroke, with my D.V.L.A. licence intact, my all London green taxi driver's licence/badge was reinstated. This whole life-changing incident led to my TOTALLY UNWANTED five minutes of fame being apparently used as a driver-retraining video in the Channel Islands also featuring in taxi trade papers, all my locals and some of the nationals.

BUSINESS AS USUAL

In late March 2004 my normal licence was re-instated by the D.V.L.A whilst I had to wait until the second week of August that year after loads of frustrating paperwork before my green London taxi badge was returned. However there was no big presentation with trumpet fanfare accompanied by cheerleaders, even though it was a massive thing to me – the only request was that both the driver and vehicle were fit to drive the public around.

This was still of a great surprise to me as the infra-red control on the steering wheel was certainly a one-off and was given a strict inspection before the Public Carriage Office would grant me a plate (a passing certificate similar to an M.O.T.) which is displayed on the back of all licensed London cabs.

On my return to work I was advised to work just a couple of hours a day in my local area. Initially it took time getting used to dealing with passengers again which at the time I found a bit strange as the infra-red control was causing a bit of a stir – many of the public are a lot more observant than you might think.

Most of my passengers now were pre-booked radio jobs using Taxi cards (the first £10.80 of the fare paid by the local authority). This was a bit different to my old days mainly up west but there was one that stood out.

SECURICAB

My first radio job one lunch time was to pick up from Snaresbrook Crown Court. On arrival at the building there was the normal array of well turned out legal types loitering around, carrying leather document cases, not an uncommon sight around Snaresbrook.

Parking as near as possible and awaiting my passenger to approach with the request of chambers in Holborn or Lincolns Inn, it came as a bit of a surprise when a security guard walked up to the cab with a passenger list instructing me to the back of the building.

Having followed his strict orders and making my way to some isolated rear doors out they marched two stern looking female guards with a tired looking waif of a girl, probably early twenties, handcuffed to one of them.

All three of them settled on the back seat with the chained girl securely positioned in the middle; there was no need for me to ask for a destination as their uniforms spoke volumes "Holloway Prison please, driver, quickest route and no hanging about."

You just get a vibe of some passengers but trying to spark up any kind of conversation would have been out of the question as I could just sense this girl was not on trial for nicking cds out of Woolworths.

It didn't take me too long to get back in the swing of things mainly working locally. However I was soon back watching Chelsea, home and away, and out and about with my old local motley crew drinking.

Work wise and socially I thought I could carry on regardless.

Part 4

Life is a Roller Coaster

This is the one chapter I so wish I didn't have to write.

Pre-Christmas 2004 four of my friends, having parked their car in my garden, set off for a sunny winter break on the beaches of Thailand from where two of them, John and Tracey Andrews, never returned having died in the cruel Boxing Day tsunami.

After the dreadful period of late 2004 early 2005 my life seemed to be like some crazy fairground ride and full of unexpected dips.

There was the odd high especially when on April 30th 2005 I was fortunate enough to be in the Reebok stadium in Bolton to see Chelsea win the league title for the first time in fifty years.

As the summer approached I was looking forward to an outing myself and some of the boys had been attending the last few years racing at Ascot this summer; due to the course being under repair, the meeting had been moved to York.

This location still suited as some of the lads lived in Derbyshire.

Thursday 16th June, having boarded a morning train from St Pancras to Derby, my pal Ian picked me up at the station taking me to stay at the family home where Ian's wife Jill and children made me extremely welcome as always.

Up early the next morning, suited and booted, following a good home-cooked breakfast we were picked up for an early train from Derby to York.

By now my old sense of direction was getting back to normal, although perhaps not quite pre-stroke, but we seemed to be heading away from Derby station and into the countryside. All of a sudden we pulled into a remote field where we were faced with the strange but welcoming sight of some of Ian's pals – good lads who I already knew – standing beside a helicopter.

We all said our hello's and I gathered this to be their transport to the races; being completely taken aback whilst awaiting my lift back to the station I was also handed a champagne flute and invited to board for the air journey as well.

Having arrived in style, what a weekend – can't remember backing any winners, just enjoyed a thoroughly special time as the lads took me on a tour of the north's lively nightlife taking in York Leeds and Blackpool.

Sunday afternoon was time to get back to normal; caught the train back to St Pancras, made my way home to Woodford where I stayed at my parents' house. That night a deep sleep was disturbed by crazy dreams of being on the floor surrounded by green uniforms and Doctor Martin shoes, but all of a sudden reality started to sink in as I realised there was a paramedic explaining that he was going to wipe the blood away from my face and try to fit breathing apparatus as I had crashed out of bed and through the bedside table.

The next thing I remember was being informed that I had been rushed into A&E, was still a bit hazy and thinking that my mum had gone over the top for a small nose bleed.

Having been kept in overnight when the consultant came around for his morning visit he informed me that when the paramedics arrived at my house they thought I was having some kind of fit or seizure (incorrect diagnosis of course!).

Once he heard my explanation of what I had been up to that weekend his conclusion was that any fit/seizure could have been caused by a combination of partying too hard, lack of sleep and maybe the helicopter ride still really properly unproven to this day.

Having been released as soon as possible I booked an appointment with my original Queen Square Neurology Hospital consultant who explained after liaising with the A&E consultant and my own G.P. that from the stroke there may be a small brain tear causing epileptic seizures and prescribed anti-convulsing medication – at the time I didn't understand the full implications of this.

Driving Licence Revoked One Year – Part Two:

ANOTHER TWIST IN THE TALE

Acceptance was the order of the day again as my annual follow-up appointment arrived in the Queen Square Neurology Hospital.

At this point my consultant explained, "Ian, you have developed epilepsy – meaning the wiring of your brain sometimes goes haywire, causing blackouts. Even though we have prescribed medication, this is not something that will just go away and you have to be careful as this loss of consciousness could be potentially dangerous."

Initially I probably took this diagnosis a little too lightly, thinking it was okay just to carry on as normal, whilst one morning another fit occurred when travelling on a fairly empty tube train. Prior to this seizure a weird buzzing noise started in my left ear so I did get a warning; luckily for me another passenger saw me slide down the seat and phoned for an ambulance who took me to A&E from where I was released that afternoon.

2005 drifted into 2006 which for me was a tame period, the main high points being in attendance at Stamford

Bridge as Chelsea won the title for the second year running whilst the D.V.L.A. returned my driving licence with all the original groups intact, especially my full motorcycle entitlement – all ready for my next venture.

BLACK AND WHITE FILM IMPERSONATORS, IMPULSIVE PURCHASE

2007 was time for me to get my show back on the road with perhaps an occupational change of direction.

Mid-2006 I had started renting my taxi out as my medical history did not yet cover me to be licensed for hire and reward (passenger cover insurance); removing the infra-red module was not a big deal as it might sound, only being attached by a standard nut and bolt.

With this first taxi on the road, grand ideas loomed of buying more and running a whole fleet.

Second on my agenda although having only dabbled whilst training to be a cabbie all those years ago, I always thought by using my knowledge of London I could earn a living as a motorcycle despatch rider. Faced with two major obstacles it was time to put my plan into action and overcome the following problems.

Firstly I had no motorcycle.

Secondly did I still have the relevant skills to ride one after so long?

Around by my house there was a regular flow of learner motorcyclists being taken through their paces by instructors as I live on a test route. One morning having managed to snatch a quick word with one of these instructors, whilst not boring him with the full history of all my health issues, he came up with the following suggestion: "you are bound to be a bit rusty, why don't you see if you can still ride a pushbike as balance is the name of the game."

Luckily for me a friend had a spare mountain bike in his garage; but don't believe the old saying "it's just like riding a pushbike" – having not ridden one for over thirty years I was all over the place just like a character from those old black and white films.

Much to the delight of my pal his pushbike was returned in one piece but still my mind was made up and, not being one for rational thinking, it was time for action.

Courier bikes in town have a tendency to fall into two categories – let's just say older well-worn ones or pristine top-of-the-range smart latest flagships with full luggage capacity whilst the riders sport smart waistcoats advertising their employees' logo.

Around London a rare-looking machine had appeared which had my name written all over it – Piaggio were taking Europe by storm with a three-wheeled road scooter which they advertised and I quote "offers unrivalled stability on wet or loose tarmac" – what more could I ask for.

My local library helped me to search the internet (still alien to this eighties throwback) where we came upon a dealer in Watford who could supply this new kind of bike.

Of course I had to pay them a visit and was most impressed with what was on show, whilst the owner could not have been more helpful, quickly summoning his workshop to assure me that the slight left-hand side modifications which would have to be carried out on the hand controls were not a problem as also this scooter is a twist-and-go with no clutch.

A test ride was out of the question, hence I headed off home doing my calculations on a British rail napkin.

Following a further visit to Watford to tie up the loose ends, two weeks later my m.p.3. 400 with modified left-handed controls was delivered by van to my garage at my home.

The anticipation was at fever pitch; when I had spoken to the instructor from the motorcycle school he explained that pupils start off in a school playground, usually on the school's own bikes before being taken on the road.

Having booked lessons and found a firm who could relay my bike, on arrival at the playground I am sure as the other pupils stood nervously beside their school 125cc bikes with L plates they must have thought look at CHARLIE BIG as the huge scooter was wheeled out the back of the van.

Each rider's lesson begins with an instructor walking backwards in front of you as you navigate figure of eights through traffic cones and I didn't look so clever as I hit a fair few.

For someone who had ridden a fully-laden motorbike up the east coast of Australia, having to dodge all sorts of wildlife and also across Europe, this was quite hard to accept.

Therefore it was back on the van and home, with the school stating that I was perhaps not ready for the road part yet – but not to give up hope – they were great as motorcycle and scooter types always seem to be full of encouragement whilst putting your safety first.

Another avenue had to be examined even though my full driving licence had been returned with full motorcycle groups reinstated I decided to finance myself for another test at the Queen Elizabeth Foundation.

With all the necessary medical checks having been carried out, on arrival at the centre having explained my latest targets the Q.E.F. staff explained to me that they did not really deal with scooters but I would have to complete the whole driving test again – private track, eyesight, memory, reactions, static rig and of course on the road.

To my delight they still considered me fit to drive a car but with a spinner attached to the steering wheel. However it was their advice to be extremely careful although legal before taking to the road on two wheels but hopefully one day I will.

Overall my latest purchase proved to be an ill thought out impulsive scheme.

HIGHS AND LOWS

Early in 2008 my emerging London taxi fleet grew (well, a second one was added and rented out), whilst the m.p.3. scooter became a permanent fixture undercover in my garage.

On the football front, since Chelsea had enjoyed two memorable title successes in 2005 and 2006, Manchester United had wrestled the title back for the last two years.

With the two clubs contesting the European Champions League final in Moscow in 2008 this is of course the height of club football and I had to be in attendance.

But sadly, for those of us who made that long journey, Chelsea lost in a penalty shoot-out, having suffered a similar experience twice before when England lost in Italy in the World Cup in 1990 and at Wembley at Euro '96 – I was also in the ground for both of these games, I am starting to think I am a jinx.

My next trip soon came around as mid-June I headed off with some mates to join 50,000 other revellers at the Isle of Wight music festival for the weekend; this was a real trip back to my youth when the Sex Pistols took to the stage and belted out some old favourites.

Whilst headlining Sunday night and closing the festival, what a treat as thousands of air guitars appeared with all ages standing side by side fully taking up Sting's offer to join in especially with an unforgettable encore of ROXANNE (which must have been heard on the mainland). It doesn't get much more nostalgic than that, the original Police line-up.

There was one more outing to be planned for this year when I attended my friends Jim and Monica's wedding celebrations in Poland. Monica is Polish and her family made all of us extremely welcome and certainly knew how to throw a party, and all of us who travelled over from Britain had a great time.

However, never count your chickens – although it had been a fairly good year, one of the strangest incidents was still to come.

PLEASE REMAIN BEHIND THE YELLOW LINES

Ever since my stroke in 2003 I had carried on with physio to try and get my left hand functioning properly again, and for the last four years along with my knowledgeable and much trusted physio, Sue King and her staff using a new device named a saeboflex – this is a revolutionary new rehab device that assists neurologically impaired individuals with opening their hand for grasp and release activities that would otherwise be impossible.

On Monday 3rd of November I was invited to take part in the saebo day at the Hilton hotel in Dartford, an exhibition where the manufacturers could see how some of their clients were getting on with their product. Having caught an early train, a long day followed being put through my paces by the saebo team along with Sue, my physio, in attendance.

Having completed all the required tasks, late afternoon I made my way back to London. Upon arrival at Liverpool Street via Charing Cross the underground was in complete chaos and therefore took the second option to use the over-ground to Chingford which was now getting unusually congested but did manage to secure a seat with a couple of minutes before the train left. With fellow commuters explaining reasons for their late departures to those at home, there seemed to be mobiles blaring throughout the carriage when all of a sudden I heard that personal unwanted ringtone in my left ear and started to anticipate that a seizure may be approaching. Another passenger noticed that I was shaking and assisted me off the train for a breath of fresh air.

Next thing I was informed of aimlessly wandering down the platform but do remember tumbling off straight onto the lines, luckily for me where I landed was not electric. A passing member of the public along with the station staff really came up trumps helping me back onto safe ground and calling an ambulance who whipped me straight into the Homerton hospital for another brief stay, having broken my left arm and four metatarsals in my left foot, which of course meant two months in plaster and out of action again.

Driving Licence Revoked One Year – Part Three.

TWO CABS, ONE SCOOTER AND THREE AMBULANCES

For the last three years I had been in complete denial about my latest neurological situation, although family knew my explanation to friends was even though having been totally sober at the time it's quite normal to fall asleep on your feet whilst walking down Liverpool Street platform and tumble on the lines (as you do).

Once my plaster had been removed in January 2009 and now left with a noticeable left-sided limp it didn't take me long to get back on full throttle behaviour.

Monday March 23rd, having been on a bit of a weekend bender, popped into one of my old locals early evening before going round to my parents' house but completely out of the blue with no warning whatsoever a fit occurred (this is the biggest regret of my life what I have put them through seeing me go into seizure mode, especially when self-inflicted).

Realising this was a major one, and on the ball as always, the relevant call was made.

When the first emergency vehicle turned up the paramedics realised to bring this seizure under control a special injection was needed, which for some reason they were unable to carry out, immediately summoning further assistance which I was told to be a routine ambulance – hopefully without screaming blue lights – quickly followed by a third emergency response vehicle seconds behind which was carrying the required serum and administered the injection.

This must have been like a scene from a horror movie set. By now some of the neighbours were getting a bit concerned; my parents had lived in the same house for thirty years and usually kept themselves to themselves but looking back I had certainly had my moments.

When first passing out as a cab driver the first cab I rented wouldn't start one day and the garage turned up with a spare one plus another to charge the flat one off, whilst nowadays the m.p.3. scooter had been stored in my dad's garage constantly being transported backwards and forwards by van.

The neighbours must have thought he's up to his old tricks – whatever next!

DECISION TIME

Following another night in A&E, awoke the next morning looking up at the gleaming white ceiling with the now familiar smell of hospitals I asked myself "is this my life, a couple of times a year I end up in here?" As we went through the routine I was now so used to, the consultants' morning round, an impressive looking female consultant, starched white coat with stethoscope casually draped around her neck and perfectly positioned under the lapels, remarked "although under control from medication these fits only seem to occur when alcohol is leaving your system."

This may well prove to be the turning point of my life as I promised myself that I would never drink again, an agreement that had been broken on numerous occasions before and a pact that every drinker has made with themselves.

NO NEED TO SIGN THE Q.E.F. VISITORS BOOK

From March onwards, 2009 was to prove to be an interesting year. Whilst attending a conference held by the Stroke Association a couple of years earlier, when chatting to one of the other guests I told her of my intentions of one day writing a book about my cab driving tales football travels and health issues.

Her advice, as she had done a fair bit of writing herself, was to join a creative writing class which I immediately enrolled on and really enjoyed at my local community centre; however when handing in my hand-written assignments it was quickly brought to my attention that they really needed to be typed out which meant using the dreaded computer.

A trip to my local library soon eased these doubts and within ten weeks, plus a second thirteen-week course at an adult education centre, a couple of basic pass certificates were achieved (hark at me).

On the football front, still being a regular at Chelsea as they won the F.A. cup again by defeating Everton at Wembley.

December 2009, once again I financed myself for another driving retest at the Queen Elizabeth Foundation where on arrival being greeted by two examiners whom I had not seen before with them remarking "you probably know the procedure as well as us."

Having satisfied their requirements for eyesight perceptual skills, static rig and of course the centre's own track whilst it had already been explained to me that due to not having a licence it was impossible to go on the public road, their recommended procedure was to apply to the D.V.L.A. for my licence along with today's Q.E.F. centre report which again would advise having a steering control spinner attached to the steering wheel and to make my application in January 2010.

This year the recession had really started to bite, resulting in earlier in the year the garage who were carrying out repairs and finding drivers to rent my cabs informing me that they could no longer make this arrangement pay, advising me to sell them. Even though I tried to find my own drivers by advertising in the taxi trade press, this proved a very awkward task and a lot more difficult to build up your own small fleet than I ever imagined.

As for the m.p.3. scooter, that certainly had to go where I never used the old favourite; one elderly lady owner claiming in the 'for sale ad' delivery mileage only was not misleading, but finally selling it to one of east London's major dealers who was quite surprised when being handed the original left-sided indicator switch which had been removed for modification and luckily for me picked the machine up by van.

If I had held on any longer, the loss on my vehicle collection would have been huge but maybe this provided funds for a future project.

CAN A LEOPARD CHANGE ITS SPOTS?

2010 started off with a weird incident as whilst knocking tiles off the wall in the bathroom at my flat another fit occurred but after a quick couple of hours in A&E this was described as a one-off virus.

As soon as possible this was explained to the D.V.L.A. as along with new licence application and last Q.E.F. report again I was informed that my latest application would take another year.

It had been a major disappointment when my brief flirtation with being a taxi proprietor had not worked out, but not as big a blow as seeing my m.p.3. scooter disappear over the horizon.

Well these things happen and I had to start planning again for my next scheme; it was time to join the electric car/scooter revolution for hopefully next year with a g-wiz car being high on the list or one of the few electric scooters which always seem to be the next great thing, having checked out all the charging points and special electric parking bays in central London.

But I am determined to think this one through – not like the m.p.3. scooter.

On the social front things were looking good as Chelsea secured the domestic double (league and F.A. cup) for the first and what will probably be the only time in our history where I was in attendance for most games and the final at Wembley whilst parading both trophies in the Kings Road on Sunday May 16th. As the champagne flowed on these unforgettable occasions, at no time was I in the slightest bit tempted to indulge.

The Isle of Wight music festival provided the next big outing of the year where my favourite band opened – Squeeze – but not on the main stage only in a side tent; there was a real treat in a tent known as the big top on the second night as an old favourite Suzi Quatro really rolled back the years with a superb set.

My year ended with my annual appointment at the Queen Square Neurology hospital where my consultant reached an important decision – ever since my first epileptic seizure in 2005 I have been taking anti-convulsing medication, every year trying to get the dosage reduced it came as a huge disappointment when my consultant informed me this type of medication would be required for life.

Whilst it is the strict rules of the Public Carriage Office who run the London taxi trade that in order to be licensed to hold a green badge and carry passengers you must be free of this type of medication for ten years.

Therefore it does not take a mathematical genius to figure out my position on that one.

MEDICAL ALERT BRACELET TAKES PREFERENCE OVER ELECTRIC CAR

Having again completed all the relevant forms once medically cleared, my D.V.L.A. driving licence was returned by post starting on January 19th 2011; by now the electric car hunt was in full flow (although luckily cheque book had remained fastened in pocket).

On January 22nd whilst attending my late friend Kevin Shipsey's yearly memorial dinner, in front of Kev's family and some good friends felt that awful left-sided numb head coming on and started to shake (no there had not been any alcohol involved).

This resulted in good pal Paul Adams jumping in a cab with me before the first course to make sure I got home, from where an ambulance was called resulting in another night spent as an inpatient.

Feeling dreadful about the whole incident of perhaps spoiling the evening for everyone and starting to think that I was becoming a bit of a liability, realised it was time to come out of the woodwork.

A couple of days later joining the epilepsy society who have certainly made me a lot more aware of this condition, in their first magazine I received one of the columnists who writes superb articles (tonic comic) brought to my attention a medical alert bracelet that most paramedics would be aware of, attached with a discrete locket enclosing waterproof information of the wearer's condition.

Investing in one of these bracelets and joining the epilepsy society may prove to be a wise investment; mid-October even being in attendance at the society's annual conference in London which really proved to be a wealth of information.

Socially 2011 was fairly low-key, gave the Isle of Wight festival a miss coming to realise that isolating myself in a tent for three days is perhaps not the best of ideas, along with long-haul flights.

However, Ian tours still continue – at the moment writing this chapter on my new favourite form of travel – the Eurostar – returning from a match at Genk in Belgium where Chelsea drew instead of getting the win they desperately needed.

THERE WILL NEVER BE ANOTHER TONIGHT

2012 starts quietly, hoping it's going to stay that way.

On the football front, after a disappointing league season another good day out is had at Wembley as Chelsea defeat Liverpool to win the F.A. cup for the seventh time having already qualified against all odds for the champion's league final against Bayern Munich to be played in the Bavarian's own Allianz Arena in Munich on May 19th, making us huge underdogs.

With an early morning cab booked on May 18th, off I head to Gatwick; on arrival in Munich make my way to my hotel by using the efficient underground system to my destination about twenty minutes outside central Munich, getting well settled in ready for the big day.

SATURDAY MAY 19TH, MATCH DAY

Get up early for a continental breakfast but as the game is an evening kick-off this leaves a day to kill for a bit of sightseeing, not like the old days when my time would have been spent traipsing around the many Munich beer halls, there is only one thing on my agenda – the B.M.W. motorcycle showrooms, as I still keep my eyes on the scooter press it has not escaped my notice that B.M.W. are about to enter the scooter market so off to their impressive exhibition centre I go.

Amongst the superb range of luxury touring machines there it stands, the new pristine 600cc road scooter. Of course enquiries have to be made from the immaculately turned out salesgirl concerning import procedure (dream on, Ian, could have ended up positioned side-by-side in your garage with the three-wheeled mp3 scooter you never rode, if you had kept it).

After a good day, back to the hotel shower and shave, light evening meal returning back into central Munich again where the place is really buzzing, make my way out to the amazing Allianz Arena stadium and take my seat half an hour before kick-off; although there is supposed to be a fifty/fifty split of tickets in the ground, understandably the home fans seem to have a larger allocation.

Having said hello to a few pals, I get settled in and must admit it is a nostalgic moment as the sound system belts out the Chelsea anthem The Liquidator by Harry J All Stars and I feel privileged to be here (not that I am wearing club colours or ever been one for singing) but really feel it doesn't get much better than this.

Kick-off arrives with the game being played at a frantic pace, Chelsea are really on the back foot and Munich should have finished the game off with that looking to be the case when in the eighty-third minute they take the lead, leading up to an unbelievable set of consequences as Chelsea striker Didier Drogba heads home an eighty-eighth minute equaliser to take the game into extra time.

Extra time is played out, with no more goals and somehow the long drawn out battle is taken to a penalty shoot-out.

In a real edge of the seat nerve-racking finale, Didier Drogba steps up to slot the fifth and final winning penalty home.

**CROWNING CHAMPIONS OF EUROPE
CHELSEA F.C.**

Following mass celebrations in the stadium, the Chelsea fans headed back into central Munich in a real party mood.

This was probably the best night of my life, when I arrived back in my room that night I looked into the mirror and realised I was talking to myself when I said:

"THERE WILL NEVER BE ANOTHER TONIGHT."

Perhaps my own life and the route of my chosen football team have followed parallel paths, one hell of a bumpy ride with loads of ups and downs thrown in.

ADAPTING TO CHANGE/CONCLUSION

Ever since March 2003 there have been major changes to my life both physically and mentally although now impatient and sometimes bad tempered perhaps having to accept (it is what it is) but there were those of a positive nature around 2008/9 I finally got to resume some sort of gym activities of course there were no more high activity circuit classes for me as I could no longer run, whilst my left hand grip and overall balance will always be impaired.

However after consulting with my doctor and consultant their advice was to try finding a low impact exercise supervised class. Therefore after a quick bit of research it was brought to my attention that the original gym where my stroke occurred runs just the thing a recovery class which is extremely well run by a couple of instructors who are most knowledgeable in training people returning form injury and illness with perhaps long time health conditions.

Also pre stroke I had always been a keen swimmer an activity which one day I hoped to return to, the recovery group had an aqua class as well. Having informed the instructor of my epilepsy enrolment was encouraged to this class, aqua class entails carrying out aerobic exercises in the shallow end of the pool my favourite being the use of light polystyrene dumb bells, hopefully joining in these classes is proving beneficial.

Many of the members in these groups are probably fifteen to twenty years older than me and have to be admired for their perseverance and efforts (but it came as a bit of a shock when one of the staff enquired if she could put my name down for the seniors Christmas party I couldn't really see myself wearing a paper hat singing carols), as when attending Chelsea matches home and abroad for forty years I have never joined in the singing.

Lucky 13

March 24th 2016 marks a huge personal milestone for me the thirteenth anniversary since suffering a stroke.

Of course I realise how extremely lucky I have been whilst perhaps having to accept that I will always have a slight left sided mobility problem.

On the epilepsy front, coming to terms with the stigma of this now realizing that by not overdoing things and keeping my medication under control a seizure will always be a risk.

This date is also seven years to the day since a drink passed my lips (without ever having been tempted.)

FINALLY

This knight of the road who once road a motorbike up the east coast of Australia and partway across Europe whilst earning his living as a London taxi driver is now a knight of public transport who no longer drivers, fully coming to terms with the fact that my cab badge has been taken forever.

THAT'S MY ADVENTURE
IT'S BEEN ONE HELL OF A RIDE OH
WEL, ONWARDS AND UPWARDS
LET'S SEE WHAT'S NEXT
THANKS FOR READING

IAN

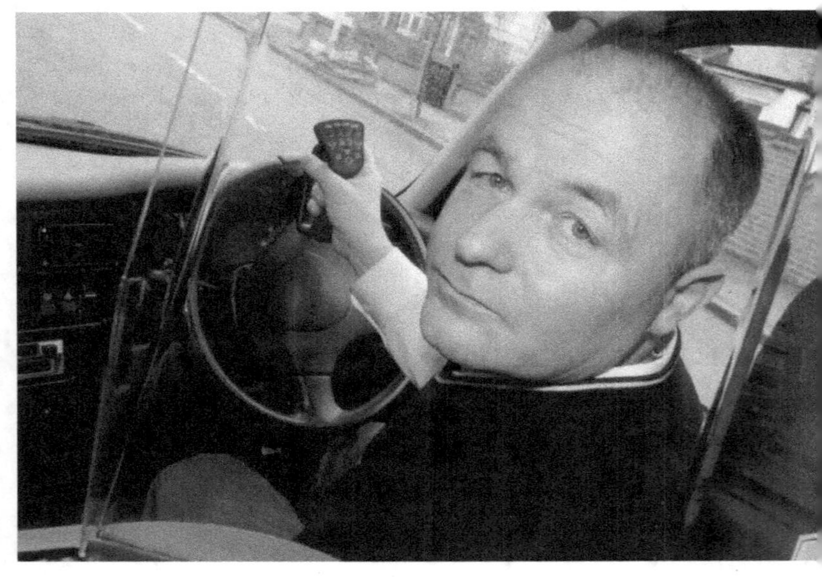

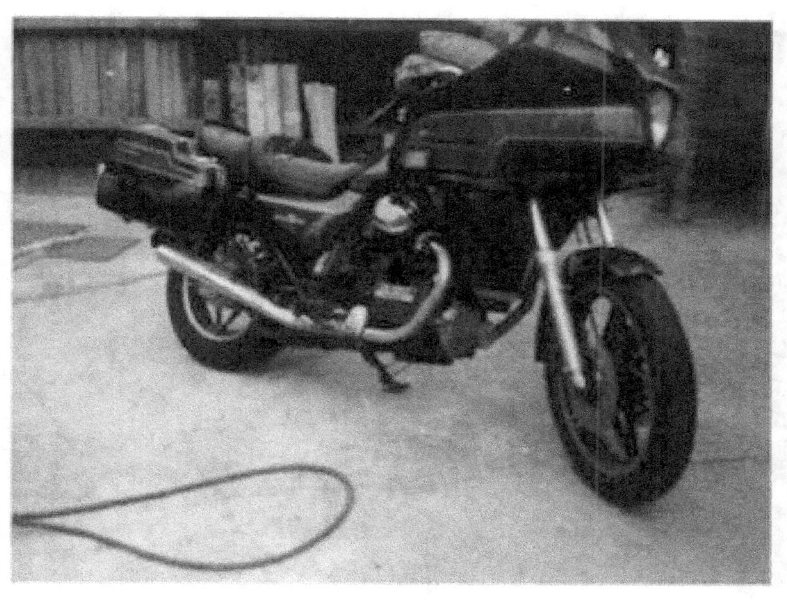

Maroon Silverwing

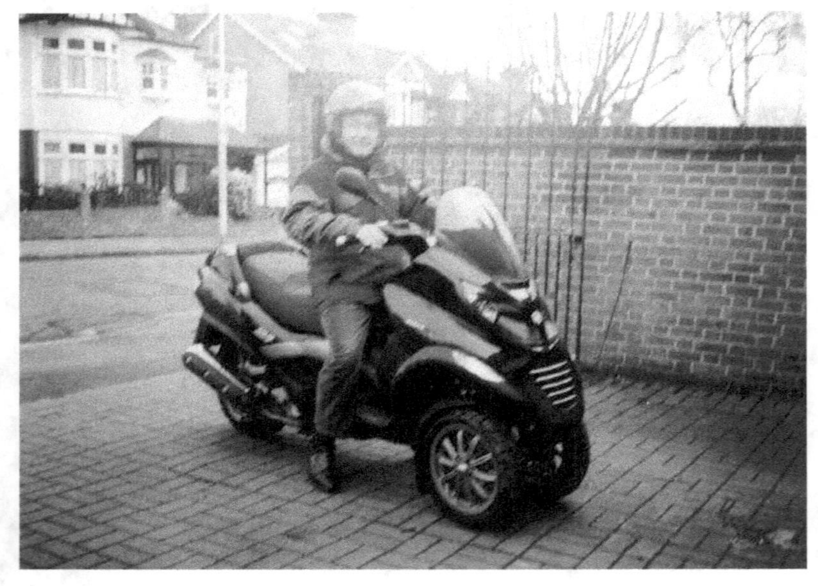

Blue three-wheeled scooter

Last Updated: Saturday, 23 April 2005, 23:58 GMT 00:58 UK

E-mail this to a friend   Printable version

'I didn't think I'd drive my cab again'

By Jane Elliott
BBC News health reporter

Taxi driver Ian Starkey thought his career was at an end when he was forced to hand in his badge following a stroke.

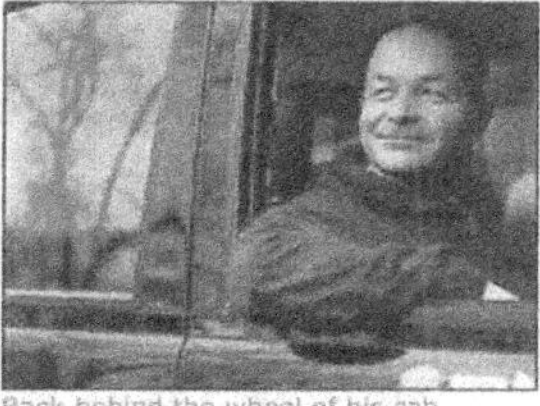
Back behind the wheel of his cab

But a special driving centre not only got him back on the road, but also driving his cab within 17 months.

Ian, of South Woodford, London, was always fit and active. He skied and regularly attended his local gym.

So when he fell on the slopes during a skiing break in France, he thought nothing of it.

Fall

Once home he went back to the gym and fell over while doing circuit training. He was unconscious and the gym instructor called an ambulance.

"They told me I had had a stroke. I had never been ill before," he said.

He was left with paralysis on his left-hand side, slightly slurred speech and a damaged left leg.

> **I thought my life as a cabbie was over at just 40**
> Ian Starkey

Ian spent two months in hospital receiving rehabilitation care and built up a good rapport with his occupational therapist, who even went with him to hand in his badge to the Public Carriage Office.

"I thought my life as a cabbie was over at just 40," Ian said. He had to give up his cab licence for a year.

However, his occupational therapist told him about the Queen Elizabeth Mobility Centre, which provides an extensive training programme for people with disabilities who want to learn or re-learn to drive.

They advised Ian to have his car fitted with infra-red controls to control anything normally done by the left-hand side of his body and allow him to do one-handed steering.

Continued...

"When I went there it was amazing. They have loads of
adapted cars so, if you cannot use your left or right-hand
side, you can still drive.

"Everyone was really surprised I was driving again. It was
easier than I expected to get behind the wheel, but I do not
do as many hours as I used to."

He applied for a new licence from the DVLA to drive a
specially adapted car and, after a doctor's report, nine
minutes on the treadmill at the hospital, and the report from
the motability centre, he was declared fit to drive his taxi
again and got his badge back.

Rehabilitation

Geraldine Dunne, of the Queen Elizabeth Foundation Mobility
Centre, said that while it was a positive outcome for some
that others were told they were not fit to drive.

"Sometimes it is not a positive outcome for people because
they do not have the reaction skills or the concentration to
drive."

But she said that those who were passed as fit to drive were
given a full range of tests before being allowed to drive on
the open roads.

"We do two sorts of assessments. A shorter assessment for
those with physical problems like head injuries and cerebral
palsy, or those who are missing limbs, and a longer
assessment for those with cognitive impairments."

She said some drivers might
need adaptations to their cars
such as a left foot accelerator
or a specially lightened
steering wheel.

The would-be drivers spend
some time on a static rig
designed to test their reactions
to a series of lights and their
steering wheel strength.

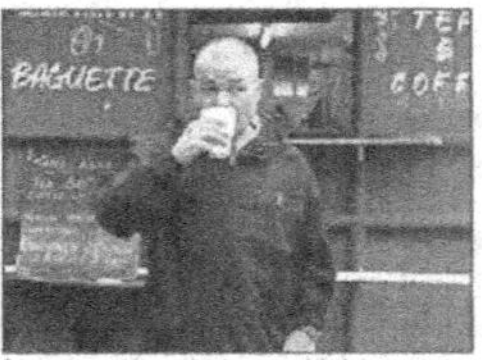

Ian never thought he would drive again

Those who pass are allowed to drive on a track at the centre
and then those who are legally able to drive on the roads are
taken out under supervised conditions.

Professor Nadina Lincoln, clinical psychologist working in
stroke rehabilitation at the University of Nottingham, said it
was important that people like Ian had stringent tests before
being allowed back on the roads.

"After a stroke people could have physical or cognitive
problems and problems with responding and thinking," she
said.

"They could have problems with spatial relationships and
might not be able to work out where a junction is.

"They might have problems judging distances or depth."

Continued...

She said that, for the first six months after a stroke, the body
had a period of recovery, so added that people were advised
not to reapply to drive before then.

"Also, during this time, people learn to adapt and
compensate for their problems."

But she said it was important that people were realistic about
their recovery, and said some people would never be fit
enough to drive again.

London Jobs/Education

The good news is

EDUCATION NOTES

Climate-change competition

THE European Commission is inviting children from EU countries, aged six to 16 years, to take part in its Green Week schools competition 2005. This year's competition highlights issues of climate change. The 20 best entries will be displayed at an exhibition in Brussels and the top three entrants will win a trip to the Belgian capital, with a parent or guardian. The deadline for entries is 15 March. Visit www. greenweek2005.eun.org

Masterclasses for IT skills

ARE you keen to improve your IT literacy skills in the classroom? The Teaching Awards Trust in London is running a series of master-classes for primary and secondary teachers called "E-Learning in an E-Confident school". Call Helen Black, 020 7776 2343/ www.teaching awards.com/training.

Tackle bullying on the net

WORRIED about bullying in

Serious illness can destroy your confidence, making a return to work extremely difficult. **Liz Bestic** asked three people about the problems they encountered

COUNCIL OFFICER HEART PATIENT

Louise Raisey is 40 and has two children, aged six and three. She lives with her husband, Kevin, in Ealing. She is a PR manager for Hammersmith and Fulham Council. Three years ago, she had open-heart surgery to correct a blocked artery. She says:

WHEN I started to get chest pains every time I ran or did any physical exercise a few months after the birth of my second child, it never occurred

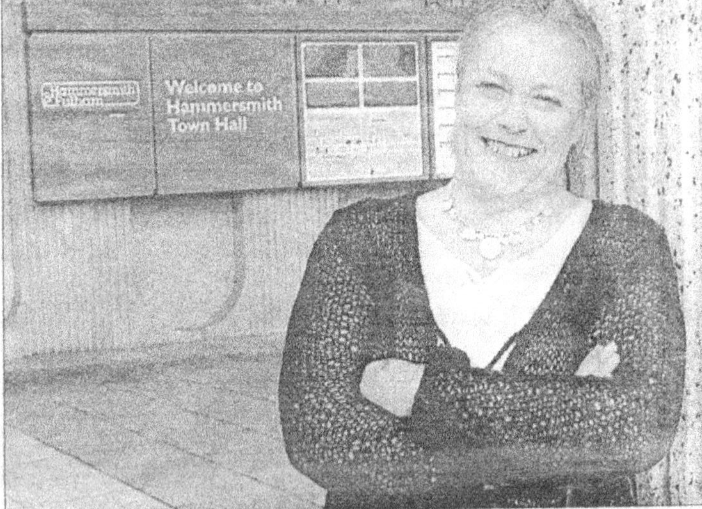

Louise Raisey: "Everyone seems to have forgotten that I have been through life-changing surgery and expects me to be back to normal"

WHERE TO STUDY..

Nutrition

King's College, London
Courses available: BSc Nutrition and Dietetics (four years): leads to both a degree in Nutrition and Dietetics and State Registration in Dietetics (SRD). Nutrition BSc (three years): prepares students to be a nutritional scientist.
When to visit: There are open days on 19 and 25 July.
Contact: Department of Nutrition and Dietetics, King's College, London, Franklin Wilkins Building, 150 Stamford Street, London, SE1 9NH (020 7848 4268), www.kcl.ac.uk/nutrdiet

Reading University
Courses available: BSc Nutrition and Food Science (three years) or BSc Nutrition and Food Science (a four-year course that includes professional training). Subjects studied include Fundamentals of Human Nutrition, Human Physiology, Cell Biology and Biochemistry.
When to visit: The next open days will be on 24 and 25 June. Pre-taster courses are held on 4-6 July.
Contact: School of Food Biosciences, PO Box 226, Whiteknights, Reading, Berks, RG6 6AP (0118 378 8700), www.food.rdg.ac.uk/teaching

thought I had contracted an infection.

When I saw my GP, he sent me to hospital, where they did tests, including an angiogram. They saw that an artery was blocked, so I was offered the choice of an angioplasty — an operation to open the artery — or a bypass. I decided on a bypass.

I was back at work within five weeks and felt great. I no longer had a blocked artery and the blood was circulating properly. I thought I had narrowly escaped death and was ready for anything.

But now, three years on, I am exhausted and stressed out. Everyone seems to have forgotten that I have been through life-changing surgery and expects me to be back to normal.

Although I work a 25-hour week, we lost our manager a year ago so I have been doing two jobs, which has been hard. I don't think there is much understanding of people who don't want to be on the career treadmill eight hours a day. If you do not want to work all the hours God sends you are seen as a bit of a problem. I am my own worst enemy because I tend to just do as I am told.

Employers need to be more flexible

when people return from life-changing crises. After my operation, my perspective on life changed. Time suddenly seemed so precious.

Kevin and I did think about moving to the West Country, but we are tied with the kids and the mortgage. I am lucky that I job-share with my husband, which means we can share the workload and childcare. Once we appoint a new manager I hope things will settle down at work.

When you come back to work people often expect you to be the same as you were before you were ill. But you do change. I have had major heart surgery — the doctors cracked my chest open and stitched a piece of extra artery around the blockage and then pinned me back up again. I may look the same on the outside but that's not the whole truth. When I get tired and stressed I need understanding.

Having this experience has made me realise the meaning of "quality time". I used to worry endlessly about where I was going in my career and whether

'When you come back, people expect you to be the same as before'

I could keep this or that deadline. Now I think there are far more important things in life, such as playing with my children or visiting my family. I spend a lot more time doing things that I enjoy than I ever used to.

NEWSCASTER CANCER PATIENT

ITN newscaster Nicholas Owen is 58 and a familiar face on our TV screens. He lives in Surrey with his wife, Brenda, and four children. Three years ago he was diagnosed with kidney cancer, which he describes as a "bolt out of the blue". He says:

IT WAS a terrible shock to be diagnosed with cancer. I consider myself pretty fit — I don't smoke, keep active and have an occasional drink. There was no history of kidney disease in my family.

The operation to remove a kidney is tricky and takes several hours, and it took the best part of the summer to recuperate.

Because journalists are such gossips, colleagues couldn't resist keeping me up with all the news while I was off work, which was important to

me. Office gossip is the stuff of life and it kept me in the loop.

It meant that when I finally went back to work after nine weeks I was quite well informed about what was going on. Nevertheless, going back was still tough. I went through that door feeling very peculiar and rather intimidated.

The truth is, having cancer knocks you for six. There is this sense that your world has changed forever. I insisted that I did not expect to be back on the exhausting daily news treadmill at the same pitch as before.

I think anyone who has had cancer and decides to return to work must be honest with themselves and their bosses. Almost certainly you will get tired more quickly and it will take you longer to recover from bouts of hard work.

It's important to be honest from day one and settle for a routine which is less hectic. Also make it crystal clear to colleagues what you will and won't do. You may want to work a four-day week, or stop working 12-hour shifts, or not take work home any more. Stick to your guns.

People are extremely sympathetic when you first go back to work but memories fade — bosses move on and new bosses come along who may need reminding.

Lots of people have asked me if I

▶ Continued from Page 1

voice of black urban youth", as some describe him. "I like to think my work is about teenagers living in underprivileged backgrounds wherever they come from," he says.

Creating a play for inner-city school kids presented a huge challenge. "It's a very hard thing to take a play into a school," Williams says. "You're on their turf. It's their hall. Going in there and holding their attention for an hour is daunting. When I've watched the play with them, I watch the kids more than the play. And their attention is being held. Which is very rewarding."

His own background is inner-city working class — but the violence and despair in Slow Time are not based on personal experiences.

The youngest of four, he grew up in a single-parent West Indian household in Fulham, a boy with a vivid imagination who discovered a passion for theatre and writing at the age of 11 and pursued his dream through years of acting in bit parts while studying the craft of theatre writing.

"I had a love of story-telling even as a kid. My parents divorced when I was two, so it was just my mum, Gloria, who worked full-time as a nurse to support us. It was hard. But we never went without.

"I didn't have any personal experience of violence or drugs, nor did I offend or get into trouble. But I saw it all around me. A lot of my friends at school came from disturbed families."

The idea for Slow Time came out of research he did three years ago. "I spent time at a young offenders' insti-

'They've made one big mistake – but are we doing enough for them?'

tution, talking to the kids there. I didn't ask them why they were there. But the fact that they were so young, just 14 or 15 and already locked up left a strong impression on me.

"My view is that they're young, maybe they've made one big mistake, of course we should punish them — but are we doing enough for them? Kids leaving these places wind up re-

offending within six months. So you have to say: are these places really working?"

Lisa Bloom, 33, is head of drama at Bethnal Green technical college, where she has taught for two years. Slow Time was performed there recently to an audience of 180 pupils.

"The kids were transfixed," she says. "Eighty-five per cent of our kids are from a Bengali background. Most had never been to a theatre or seen a production before. They thought a play might be something they didn't understand. But because the play is very much in their language, and dealt with issues that are commonplace in this area, they really related to it.

"A lot of them weren't even aware that if you offend, you can wind up in a young offenders' institution at 10 — most thought you had to be 18. So they

London Jobs/Health

I'm going back to work

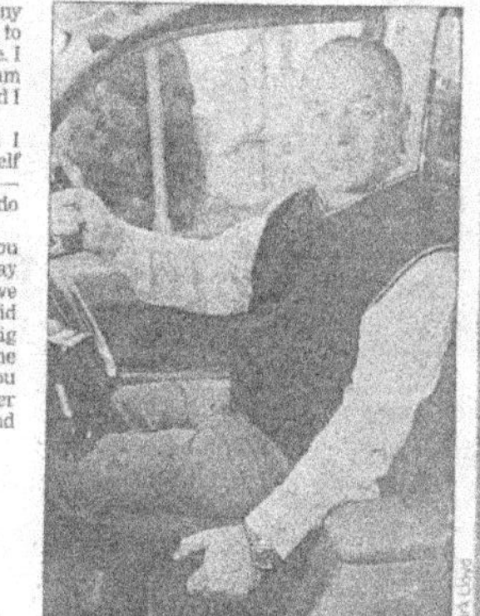

felt like giving up work after this and many people recovering from cancer decide to spend more time doing things that they love. I like golf, but my real passion is my work. I am lucky enough to have a career that I love and I am busier now than I have ever been.

I used to travel around the world and I wouldn't think twice, but now I put myself first. There are no guarantees with cancer — you have to live every day to the full and do the things that make you happy.

My message is: don't bite off more than you can chew. People who have had cancer may think they have to work twice as hard to prove they are up to the job. Some may be afraid they won't be able to cope. If you are in a big corporation where you are going up the career ladder you may have to accept you have slipped a few rungs. But if cancer teaches you nothing else it's what is and what's not important in your life.

CABBIE
STROKE PATIENT

Ian Starkey is 43 and has been a London cabbie for 15 years. Two years ago he was at a gym when he tripped on the running machine. The next thing he knew he was in hospital. He had suffered a stroke which affected his left side. He says:

WHEN the doctors told me I had had a stroke I couldn't believe it . There is no history of it in my family and I had always been perfectly fit. I loved my job and the freedom it gave me — I used to work eight to 10 hours a day, five days a week. Suddenly I was lying in a hospital bed wondering if I would ever be able to work

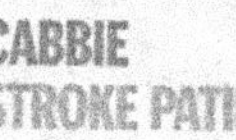

On the road again: cabbie and stroke patient Ian Starkey

the all-clear to drive an adapted vehicle. The Mobility Centre then gave me the name of a company who could adapt my cab.

My next task was to prove to the London Carriage Office that I was fit enough to drive people around. I couldn't believe it when they said "Yes" and gave me back my precious green badge!

In many ways going back to work has been like starting out as a cabbie all over again. I

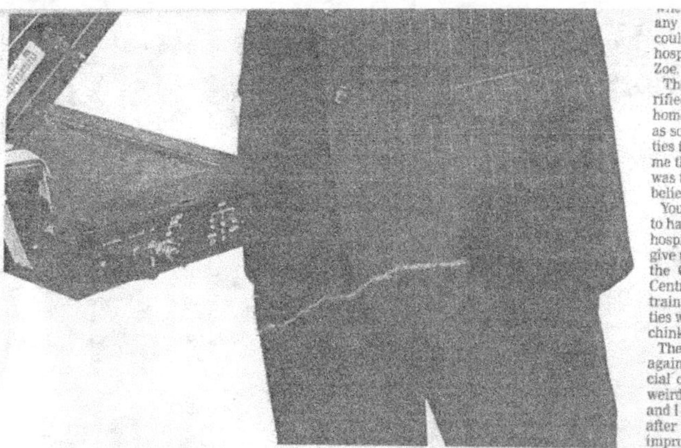

...wheelchair for a week because I couldn't put any weight on my left leg, and I don't think I could have got through those two months in hospital without my occupational therapist, Zoe.

The thought of what lay in store for me terrified me. I knew the bills were piling up at home and I had to be able to get back to work as soon as I could. Zoe had to tell the authorities that I had had a stroke and she came with me the day I had to hand back my badge. That was the hardest thing I ever had to do. I really believed my life as a cabbie was over.

You never think something like this is going to happen to you and two months of lying in a hospital bed were almost enough to make me give up and end it all. When Zoe told me about the Queen Elizabeth's Foundation Mobility Centre in Banstead, Surrey, which runs a training programme for people with disabilities who want to re-learn to drive, I could see a chink of light at the end of the tunnel.

The first time I got into the driving seat again was in a Nissan Micra fitted with special controls for one-handed steering. It was weird getting used to a new way of driving and I found myself veering off to the side. But after that first lesson I felt I had really improved. After one more lesson I was given

rather spend time skiing with my mates, and last week I went to Barcelona to watch football.

The whole experience makes you realise that your life can be snuffed out in an instant. It also makes you realise who is important in your life. I couldn't have got through this without my parents. Getting better has been a long, hard slog and many times I have felt very frustrated because I am impatient to improve. But I am proud of the fact I have regained my independence and my livelihood within 17 months of having a stroke.

A question of lost confidence

RESEARCH by the charity Cancer BACUP shows 30 per cent of people returning to work after cancer have lost confidence in their ability to do their job. The charity wants senior managers to recognise the importance of flexible working, return-to-work policies and high-quality information and support.
www.cancerbacup.org.uk

---

were really shocked. Yes, it was hard-hitting — at the end, the Asian boy is contemplating suicide — but the message got right through, there's no question of that."

Williams's research included spending time in Manchester exploring the world of young people living on the margins. "I hung out with some unemployed kids and talked to them about their lives, getting into trouble by fighting, living fast with drugs and drink.

"When you ask them why they do these things, they don't tell you they're depressed. It's almost as if they're enjoying what they are doing. They don't want a proper job, they're all looking for something that will help them get rich quick, have loads of money by the age of 20.

"The focus is money — and lots of it.

'They don't want a proper job, they want something to get rich quick'

Which is the way society has led young people. Teenagers now have been forced to grow up so quickly, they think everything comes very easy, you can be rich and famous in five minutes."

The bullying and peer-group pressure that the play explores are, says Williams, inextricably linked.

"They're joined at the hip. I wasn't bullied at school. I was lucky to keep away from it. But it happens in most schools; mine was no exception. I saw many kids too scared to say no to bullies even when they knew it meant they'd get into trouble. And the boys in the play have definitely been pushed the wrong way by peer-group pressure.

I wanted to show the danger of it, how easily it can trap you into doing something awful — that can mess up a young life. Hopefully, it's something the kids will discuss with their teachers afterwards."

Does he believe that access to live theatre and a hard-hitting play like this can really transform kids' perceptions? "Yes it can," he says without hesitation. "If they are tuned into the possibilities of what they can do, like I was, then a big fat YES."

The problems young people face

- In 2003/4, more than 31,000 children contacted ChildLine about bullying, an increase of 42 per cent on the previous year.

- The NSPCC estimates that between 50-60 per cent of children of all ages say they have been bullied at some stage. "Year nines are more likely to be bullied," says Alison O'Brien, the NSPCC's education adviser.

- Twenty-six per cent of young people in mainstream education have committed a crime.

- Latest Government statistics

show that almost 25 per cent of secondary school pupils truant at some stage. Truancy rates have increased by more than six per cent in the last year. Inner London has the worst rate in England, with up to 15,000 schoolchildren missing from lessons on any given day.

- Slow Time is part of NT Education's Interact project, where actors perform plays in schools using drama as a stimulus for topics like Citizenship, introduced into the secondary school curriculum in 2000. www.nationaltheatre.org.uk/edu

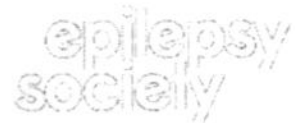

You are here: <u>Home</u> » <u>About epilepsy</u> » <u>Blog</u> » From black cabs to blackouts

From black cabs to blackouts

Created 28 October 2014

Londoner and former black cab driver Ian Starkey refuses to be beaten by a stroke which left him with reduced mobility and epilepsy. He's written a touching account of his life in a book called *From Black Cabbing to Blackouts*. This is his story...

In 2003 at the age of 40 my life came crashing down around me when a severe stroke left me with epilepsy and a weakness to the left side of my body. My 15 year career as a London cabbie was over and I realised that my life would never be the same again. However, I'm not one to sit around moping, glass half full that's me. Yes there are things I can't or shouldn't do anymore, but having the stroke has also enabled me to fulfil ambitions that may not otherwise have happened.

Writing a book

One of my greatest achievements has been writing a book. Like many people I always felt I had a book in me, the main difference is that I've stopped talking about and have committed words to paper or rather thoughts to the computer. The result is *From Black Cabbing to Blackouts* which pretty much sums up everything about me and about my life.

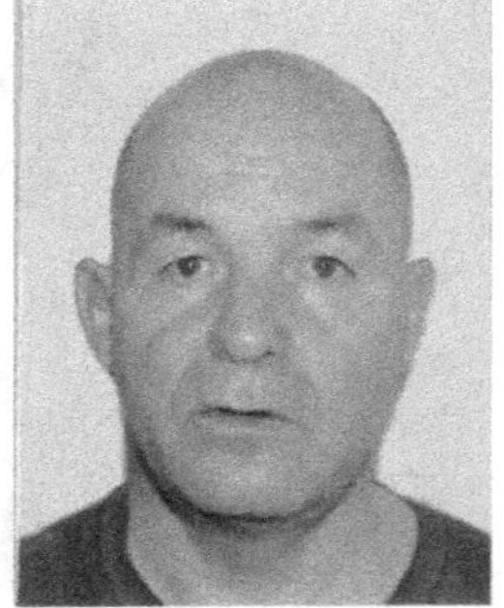

Touching on the lows, but concentrating on the highs, I was determined to document all aspects of my pre- and post-stroke life. From the dangers, tumbling off a busy commuter station platform onto a railway line during a seizure, to my pre stroke joys, travelling around the world on my motorbike and watching my beloved football team Chelsea wherever and whenever they play. Of course I'm still an avid fan and still follow the team wherever the play, however the train is my preferred mode of transport now.

Me and Freddie Mercury

There's never a dull moment in the life of a London cabbie, and yes I've had my share of well known MPs, public figures, professional sportsmen, actors and actresses in the back of my taxi, including Joan Collins and Dame Judi Dench. However the biggest surprise was when the legendary Freddie Mercury booked my cab - it doesn't get much more famous than that.

It's not all glamorous though. I had to do a pick up once from Snaresbrook Crown Court. Two stern looking female guards, handcuffed to a young tired looking waif of a girl, emerged from security doors at the back of the building. There was no need to guess where we were headed. 'Holloway Prison please driver, quickest route possible, no hanging about.' I wouldn't have wanted to strike up a conversation with their prisoner. I sensed she hadn't been on trial for nicking CDs from Woolworths.

Epilepsy stigma

It's true that I do miss elements of my former life and it's been a struggle to get back on top of things, but I've worked hard at my physio and concentrated on the positives. Last year was a milestone for me - the tenth anniversary of my stroke. I realise how extremely lucky I've been and finally accept that I'll probably always have slight left-sided mobility issues.

As far as epilepsy is concerned I'm determined to continue to fight the stigma which still surrounds this condition. I've learnt that alcohol is not my friend, I can't overdo things and I need to be careful with my medication to give myself the best chance of keeping my seizures under control.

My life so far has been one hell of a ride, I say onwards and upwards, let's see what's next.

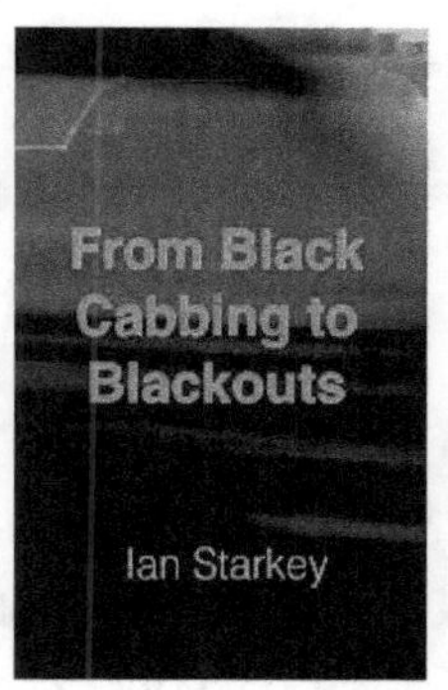

From Black Cabbing to Blackouts by Ian Starkey is available from Amazon.

Tags: ian starkey black cabs and blackouts epilepsy grand mal seizures seizures

LESSONS LEARNT AND CODE I TRY TO LIVE BY.

ITINERARY

WHAT YOU SEE IS WHAT YOU GET.

ALWAYS GO BY YOUR INSTICTS.

YOU NEVER GET A SECOND CHANCE TO MAKE A FIRST IMPRESSION.

TO FAIL TO PREPARE IS TO PREPARE TO FAIL.

AVOID LOUD ATTENTION SEEKING PEOPLE.

STAY CALM AND FOCUSED.

NEITHER A LENDER OR BORROWER BE.

YOU ONLY GET WHAT YOU PAY FOR/A FOOL AND HIS MONEY SOON PART.

OBSERVE THE GREEN CROSS CODE.

THE PAST IS NOT A TOURIST ATTRACTION TO BE VISTED AT LEISURE.

WHAT GOES AROUND COMES AROUND IT'S ALL DOWN TO KARMA.

ADVERSITY INTRODUCES US TO OURSELVES.

IF YOU PLAY THE GAME YOU KNOW THE RISKS!

ACKNOWLEDGEMENTS

Firstly, Mum & Dad

Brother Paul and partner Pauline

Nephew Keith (without your technical assistance this
    book would never have happened.)

The rest of the immediate family

To many medical people to properly thank

The excellent consultants physios and staff at
    The Queen Square Neurology Hospital

Whipps Cross Hospital

John Hines consultant urologist

All the paramedics who have scraped me off the floor

The Stroke Association

Queen Elizabeth Driving Foundation

The Epilepsy Society

Doctor Sean Howlett along with the other GPs and staff at
    Glebelands surgery

Physio Sue King/Davies and staff at Ephysio

All the pals I made in whilst driving a cab (seems a long time ago now).

Everyone I have met following Chelsea, it's been an adventure and a pleasure (with a huge thanks to Russell Lautman for all the much appreciated lifts home from Stamford Bridge over the last few years).

For patiently transferring this project onto the required format, Kate Lewis of Promoworx, South Woodford.

With a special mention to New Generation Publishing for finally getting this book on the market.

Mostly a huge thanks to all my long-time friends for trying to keep me involved over the last thirteen years.

YOU HAVE ALL BEEN GREAT!

www.ingramcontent.com/pod-product-compliance
Lightning Source LLC
Chambersburg PA
CBHW061518250726
48657CB00005B/1952